EXPLORING BORDERLINE PERSONALITY DISORDER

Progress in Just 10 Days.

Brain Training
to Master Emotions & Anxiety.

Daniel Mason

Table of Contents

INTRODUCTION 3

CHAPTER ONE: EXPLORING BORDERLINE PERSONALITY DISORDER 7

CHAPTER TWO: CAUSES OF BPD; WHO GETS BPD AND WHY? 37

CHAPTER THREE: TAKING NOTE OF THE MAJOR SYMPTOMS 73

CHAPTER FOUR: MAKING THE CHOICE TO CHANGE 91

INTRODUCTION

Individuals with borderline personality disorder (BPD) are struggling with their feelings, attitudes, and sense of identity and relationships with others. Because they are in such emotional turmoil, they frequently succumb to coping strategies that appear to be working at the moment but actually make their issues worse (such as attempts at suicide, self-harm, or substance use).

No-one knew until recently which treatments really help people with BPD. In fact, people with BPD are considered extremely frightening because they seem to have a lot of rages aimed at themselves, the people they care for, the environment, and even their doctors and therapists. Borderline rage can happen anytime and anywhere. Mental health professionals want to support their clients and help them, but people with BPD are difficult to keep healthy and often hinder the best efforts of therapists. In fact, in some way, around 75 percent of people who have BPD hurt themselves, and one out of ten succeed in suicide.

You might wonder, "Why is BPD a big topic like this now? "What took so long?" is a relevant question. People with BPD feel emotional pain that is severe. Throughout their relationships with other people, they deal with unrelenting chaos; feelings of isolation, loneliness, and desperation; and a confused sense of who they are and where they are going throughout life. In fact, up to 10 percent of BPD people commit suicide, a rate that is more than fifty times that of the general population. And, with all of this, many BPD people don't get the help they need. Individuals with BPD may have strong emotions and responsiveness that can be thrilling and intense. Those with BPD can be dramatic and enthusiastic and are often very compassionate and thorough. Nevertheless, caring for someone with BPD is like trying to hold on to the sun: a person with BPD has the emotional intensity to scorch and to char relationships. Additionally, people with BPD are often swallowed up by grief or sadness, leaving the caregiver or family member in the dark about what to do.

The most important and distinguishing feature of personality disorders, however, is the negative effect these disorders have on interpersonal relations. People with personality disorders tend to respond with a characteristically rigid constellation of thoughts, feelings, and behavior, to different situations and demands. This inflexibility and difficulty in shaping nuanced responses is the primary difference between healthy personalities and disordered. The exact cause of personality disorders is still unknown.

It is clear, however, that there are both biological and psychosocial factors influencing personality and personality disorders development.

At one time, it was thought that personality disorders were untreatable. That is not the case any more. There are now several highly effective treatments for personality disorders that stem from the same previously reviewed psychological theories. Such therapies include mentalization-based therapy (MBT), cognitive-behavioral therapy (CBT), dialectic behavioral therapy (DBT), and schema therapy, as well as pharmacotherapy.

CHAPTER ONE: EXPLORING BORDERLINE PERSONALITY DISORDER

Personality is a relatively consistent way people behave, act, perceive, and relate to others. The personality represents how others view you in general — such as calm, nervous, easily frustrated, mellow, reflective, impulsive, curious, or unapproachable. From time to time, all people differ from their usual personalities, but, for the most part, over time, personalities remain fairly stable.

A personality disorder is the other major form of psychiatric disorder. So, what is a personality disorder? The concept here is we all have conventional ways to act, smell, perceive, and respond to the environment that make up our personality. Every time you say, "He (or she) is a cool person!" Really you are referring to the personality of that person or to the typical way of behaving or relating to the environment. A personality disorder is essentially a long-lasting pattern that is not functioning very well concerning the world.

Consider, for example, someone who has a typically positive personality; this person enjoys life and people. However, when this person experiences a tragedy, you expect this generally jolly person to feel normal grief and sadness. On the other hand, someone with a personality disorder, such as BPD, encounters chronic, persistent mental, behavioral, cognitive, and/or relationship problems. Furthermore, these issues cause great distress and can create difficulties in relationships or lead to problems reaching goals in life (such as goals involving getting or maintaining the desired job). There are many different types of personality disorders, including evasive, obsessive-compulsive, dependent, paranoid, schizoid, schizotypic, narcissistic, histrionic, antisocial, and borderline personality disorder, of course. Borderline personality disorder (BPD) in the individuals it afflicts induces frustration, anxiety, and anguish. Their friends and families also suffer. BPD expresses itself as a complex mixture of long-standing patterns of thought, actions, and feelings that disrupt happiness, relationships, and productiveness. Additionally, people with this disorder have trouble controlling impulses, dealing with others, coping with emotional problems, and sometimes comprehending reality.

A BRIEF OVERVIEW OF THE HISTORY AND ROOTS OF BPD

Understanding a bit of the past of what is now called BPD is relevant. People used the word borderline in the nineteenth century to describe a condition that existed at the blurred boundary between two different types of psychiatric problems. The widely held view was that psychiatric disorders or problems existed in two broad groups. One type, called neurosis, included people who were aware of reality but had emotional problems like depression or anxiety disorders. The other group, psychosis included people who had odd thoughts and experiences (such as hallucinations) that were not based, and illnesses such as schizophrenia were diagnosed in those people. Patients that did not have issues that were sufficiently serious about being considered psychotic (i.e., their thoughts and perceptions were mostly based in reality), but were too distressed to be deemed neurotic, were placed into the category of borderline. Psychiatrists used the term borderline for people who had trouble recognizing both good and bad characteristics in humans at the same time, who lived dysfunctional and unstable lives, and who were frequently overwhelmed emotionally. Many of these ways of thinking about BPD came directly from a limited number of patients ' observations and were not based on scientific research. Researchers have led numerous studies since those early days. Findings from these researches have identified many essential characteristics that makeup what we now call borderline personality disorder, including anger control issues, impulsive behavior, and trouble with relationships and identities. People with BPD are no longer considered to border on psychosis and neurosis. Science helps us to maintain the ideas about BPD that seem to be true and to discard the old ideas about BPD that do not seem to be correct. The term "borderline" was first used more than sixty years ago to describe patients who were on the psychotic-neurotic border but could not be properly classified as either. Borderline patients behaved somewhere in between, unlike psychotic patients who were permanently divorced from reality and neurotic patients who responded more reliably to close relationships and psychotherapy. Borderlines, observed by doctors, sometimes wandered into the wild terrain of psychosis but usually remained for only a short time. Borderlines, on the other hand, displayed some superficial neurotic traits, but these comparatively healthier mechanisms of defense failed under stress.

ROOTS OF BPD

Several methodologies were used to investigate BPD's causes and roots. Family studies have confirmed that most of the borderlines have experienced severe developmental damage, leading to environmental causes. More recent genetic and neurological studies have theorized that heritable, biological underpinnings may exist. A considerable borderline subgroup has a history of perinatal or acquired brain injury. A new line of research posits that predisposing genetic/biological defects combine to create pathways for borderline coping with environmental traumas. One model suggests that hereditary tendencies (called temperament) intersect with the values (character) based on development to produce personality. It is also possible to distinguish different temperaments and to equate them with biological imbalances and sensitivities. Temperament models develop early in life and are viewed as either instinctual or habitual. Character styles are developed slowly and culminate in adulthood.

Biological and Anatomical Correlates

Some of BPD research's most exciting recent discoveries use modern medical methods to investigate brain dynamics, such as measuring chemical changes and analyzing anatomical changes. Some studies have shown that elevated levels of the neurotransmitter serotonin (a chemical that is involved in nerve conduction throughout the body but particularly in the brain) may lead to increased impulsivity and aggression associated with BPD. Surprisingly, this vulnerability is seen more often in women, who make up 75 percent of borderlines. One study used positron emission tomography (PET) scanning to show lower levels of serotonin activity in the brains of men and women with BPD, which was correlated with increased impulsiveness. Other neurotransmitters, such as dopamine and gamma-aminobutyric acid (GABA), may also be involved in regulating impulsive rage. Modulation of mood associates the neurotransmitters acetylcholine and norepinephrine. It has been shown that medicines that control these imbalances in neurotransmitters relieve borderline symptoms.

Some researchers have investigated the connection between BPD and autoimmune disorders, in which the body has a kind of allergic reaction to itself and produces antibodies to its organs themselves. Rheumatoid arthritis, for example, is associated with an unusually high BPD prevalence. A woman with fluctuating BPD symptoms followed one study over a period of nine months while her antithyroid antibodies were being measured. These investigators found significantly lower levels of the antibodies during times when their scores for depression and psychosis were low, and higher when their symptoms increased. This finding suggests that BPD symptoms may be exacerbated by autoimmune inflammation or vice versa. Scientists investigating BPD's neurology have focused on the part of the brain, called the limbic system. This brain section influences memory, thinking, emotional (such as anxiety) states, and behaviors (especially aggressive and sexual ones). EEG borderline study has shown dysfunction in this part of the brain. One study used magnetic resonance imaging (MRI) to assess changes in the volume of the limbic system in borderline women with a trauma history. Such authors showed a significant reduction in the amount of this brain area in the hippocampus and amygdala regions. This link between past physical or emotional trauma and subsequent changes in brain volume associated with borderline pathology raises the possibility that child abuse may alter brain function, contributing to borderline actions. What has not been proved definitively is the association's direction. An alternative explanation might be that BPD causes (rather than is the result of) changes in brain volume that are associated with past trauma, only fortuitously.

Over the past few years, genetic and environmental genome work has exploded. Gene mapping, cloning ability, and stem cell production have opened new frontiers in medical illness understanding and care. Some BPD researchers have tried to establish that particular types of borderline behaviors may be responsible for specific genes. For example, there are strong genetic components in identity instability, mood changes, and violent impulsivity. Another behavior frequently displayed by borderline, novelty-seeking— referring to the pursuit of excitement and sometimes danger, often to avoid feelings of emptiness and boredom — is a feature also associated with other BPD criteria, such as impulsiveness and aggression. However, several experiments in the serotonin neurotransmitter system associated this observed activity with chemical dysregulation, and other research with a gene locus affecting the dopamine neurotransmitter on a specific human chromosome. Though these studies need clarification, they indicate genetic connections, internal chemical equilibrium, and ultimately behavior. Family tests have shown that first-degree borderline relatives are five times more likely than the general public to meet the BPD diagnosis, too. Borderline family members are also more likely to be diagnosed with related diseases, notably substance abuse, affective disorders, and antisocial personality disorder. In a way, throughout one's life, those genes are "turned on and off," affected by factors such as parenting. Animal and human research evaluating maternal care indicates that positive parenting can affect genetic predisposition and biochemical equilibrium resulting from it. Thus, an individual may be born with inborn vulnerabilities to impaired brain circuitry for modulating moods and impulsivity. Still, environmental factors may affect gene expression in a manner that determines whether the person will exhibit any or all of the potential borderline symptoms.

Genetic contributions— modified by environmental influences— to the development of BPD are definitely dependent on multiple factors and likely involve multiple chromosomal loci. Nonetheless, further clarification of these mechanisms can lead to the development of new biotech drugs that can target specific genes for adaptation.

BPD's NINE SYMPTOMS

Knowing if you or someone you know has BPD requires careful evaluation and guidance from a qualified mental health professional. Many professionals struggle with making this diagnosis, however, because BPD symptoms vary dramatically from person to person. BPD is, in a way, identical to the countless dog breeds that exist today. For instance, cocker spaniels, terriers, Bernese mountain dogs, pit bulls, Russian wolfhounds, golden doodles, mutts, and chihuahuas differ markedly from each other, but they're all dogs. Similarly, people with BPD do not share the same symptoms, but all have the same disorder.

People who suffer from BPD experience a range of symptoms that are classified into nine major categories by mental health professionals. Currently, you need to show signs of at least five of these nine symptoms to be diagnosed with BPD.

1. Sensation seeking (impulsivity)

To be classified as a sign of BPD, this sensation-seeking symptom has to involve a minimum of two types of impulsive, self-destructive behaviors. Such impulsive activities cause adrenaline rushes and extreme enthusiasm. They include the following: omnipresent sexual acting out omnipresent substance abuse omnipresent spending sprees omnipresent binge eating omnipresent careless behavior, including • Extremely aggressive driving • Dangerous sports• Petty theft• Property destruction. Impulsive actions are both dangerous and self-damaging. Sometimes they endanger the lives and well-being of the people who display them. Sexual acting out, for example, may consist of regular, informal, unprotected sexual encounters with complete strangers, leading to STDs or unwanted pregnancies. Uncontained spending can involve numerous unnecessary purchases to maximize credit cards and accumulate debt. Shoplifting also involves the strict theft of things for fun and may result in jail time.

2. Self-harm

Self-harm is the most common and easily visible symptom in people with BPD. People who exhibit this symptom can and often do threaten or attempt suicide. Others can burn themselves intentionally with cigarettes, slice their arms with sharp knives, hit their heads, disfigure their skin, or even break bones in their hands or bodies. While this symptom is separate from sensation seeking, it also involves some degree of impulsiveness. People who exhibit this syndrome must be impulsive enough to try and kill themselves over and over again.

3. Roller coaster emotions

Individuals with BPD experience severe emotional swings. One moment they might feel atop the world and dive into deep despair the next. Such changes in mood are severe but typically fleeting, only lasting a few minutes or hours. The cognitive flip-flops also occur as a response to seemingly irrelevant causes. A co-worker, for example, passes someone in the hallway with BPD without recognizing her. This involuntary slight can spark powerful anxiety and distress in a BPD person. Most people in a relationship with someone who has BPD find these mood swings to be quite hard to understand or to accept.

4. Explosiveness

Dramatic outbursts of rage and anger frequently torment people with BPD. Again, the things that cause such rages may seem insignificant to others. Such explosions also wreak havoc in relationships as you can imagine, and can even result in physical confrontations. Because of their outrageous behavior, people with BPD often end up in legal chaos. Road rage is a good example of this BPD symptom, though not everyone who shows off-road rage has BPD.

5. Worries about abandonment

People who exhibit this symptom are obsessed with the fear of being left by a loved one. They can appear clingy, reliant, and outrageously jealous because of their fear over abandonment. For example, a husband with BPD can check the regular readings of his wife's cellphone logs, emails, and car odometer, often looking for evidence of infidelity. Ironically, they are usually driven away by an obsession of holding loved ones close.

6. Unclear and unstable self-concept

This symptom represents a failure to find an identity that is secure and clear. People who display this symptom may sometimes regard themselves very favorably, yet at other times they exude self-disdain. They often have little idea about what they want in life and lack a strong sense of purpose or values. Frequent changes in jobs, religion, or sexual identity can represent changing values and objectives. Navigating life without a clear concept of yourself is like trying to find your way over the ocean without any compass.

7. Emptiness

Most people with BPD report feeling empty within. They have cravings for something more, but they can't figure out what is more. They feel lonely, bored, and unfulfilled. They may try to fill their needs with shallow sex, drugs, or food, but nothing ever seems to get truly satisfying—they feel like trying to fill a black hole.

8. Up-and-down relationships

Relationships with people with BPD imitate revolving doors. Individuals with BPD often see other individuals as either good or bad, and these decisions can change from day to day or even from hour to hour. People suffering from BPD often fall quickly and intensely into love.

They put new loves on pedestals, but when the slightest deceptions (whether real or imagined) inevitably occur, their pedestals crumble. Those who have BPD in relationships (whether they are partners, co-workers, or friends) suffer mental whiplash from frequent changes from idolatry to demonization. As a result, a lot of people find it difficult to maintain meaningful relationships with those with BPD.

9. Dissociation

Feeling out of touch with reality, Professionals describe dissociation as an unreal sensation. People who feel dissociated or out of touch with reality say they feel as if they look down on themselves and see their lives unfold without being a real part of them. If people with BPD lose touch with reality, they generally for long periods do not do this. But sometimes they hear voices asking them what to do when they lose touch with reality. We may also suffer from severe, unwarranted distrust of others at certain times.

THE BORDERLINE LIFE CYCLE

Primarily, borderline behavior is first observed from the late adolescents to the early thirties, although severe separation problems or outbursts of rage in younger children can be a diagnostic harbinger. A borderline state can emerge from a parental relationship that's either too dependent or too rejecting at one of two extremes. Disruption of normal development of children, particularly during the crucial age of rapprochement (sixteen to twenty-five months), may hinder the development of a constant, separate identity, one of the prominent symptoms of BPD. Many teenagers are already dealing with problems such as personality, moodiness, impulsiveness, and uncertainty in relationships that are at the center of BPD. (Indeed, some might argue that the word ' borderline adolescent' is completely pointless!) Nevertheless, average, volatile adolescents do not exhibit suicide attempts, violent rages, or excessive drug abuse found in borderline adolescents. A lot of borderlines find some peace in their lives during their third and fourth decades. Borderline habits may be curbed or may not seriously hamper everyday activities any longer. Thus many former borderlines, with or without treatment, can emerge from the chaos of their lives to a relatively stable midlife functioning that no longer meets defining BPD diagnostic criteria. BPD occurs in the elderly but at much lower rates.

TREATMENT OF BORDERLINE PATIENT

Over the past decade, treatment for BPD has improved considerably. Specifically, controlled psychotherapy approaches and medication studies have yielded significant scientific confirmation that has done much to alleviate past pessimism. In short, Therapy works in many situations.

- *Psychotherapy*

Psychotherapy, complemented by symptom-focused pharmacotherapy, remains the cornerstone of care for BPD. At that time, evidence of the effectiveness of specific therapy techniques was based on individual case studies, rather than on controlled scientific assessments. Research comparing the efficacy of many drugs to the effects of psychotherapy have also not yet been published in the literature.

Psychotherapy refers to a wide variety of methods used to help people deal with emotional problems as well as life and relationship difficulties. The psychotherapy takes place in the context of a client-therapist partnership. Techniques include conversation, proposed changes in behavior, collection of feedback, communication, and building skills. Some of their patients receive psychotherapy from a wide range of professionals, including social workers, counselors, marriage and family therapists, physicians, psychologists, and clinical nurses.

If you have BPD, you don't just want to try any type of psychotherapy, because many psychotherapy strategies have not proven effective for this specific diagnosis. Instead, you want to get counseling based on approaches that have at least provided some empirical support for their efficacy in treating BPD.

- *Medication*

Pharmacotherapy is an important psychotherapy adjunct. Medication targets specific symptoms, especially in mood disturbance contexts, impulse dyscontrol, and perceptual distortions. The drug types used are primarily antidepressants, mood stabilizers, psychotropics (antipsychotic medications), and anti-anxiety drugs. Occasionally, ECT (electroconvulsive therapy) and opiate antagonists (which were also effective in treating self-mutilating behavior) may also be used.

Psychotropic drugs have the function of lessening or alleviating emotional pain. For many people with emotional problems prescription drugs can be life savers. In the case of BPD, however, medication does not seem to be as helpful as it is in other emotional problems. Even so, most people undergoing BPD treatment take some form of medication. And occasionally they take a surprisingly large number of medicines. Mental health professionals also offer these drugs to their patients, hoping they can reduce some of the effects of BPD in their patients. To date, however, research is only providing limited support for the usefulness of using psychotropic drugs to treat BPD.

Most individuals with BPD also have other conditions that have been effectively treated with medication, such as depression or anxiety disorders. Thus, the use of medication in people with BPD to treat other disorders can be a useful form of treatment.

COUNTING THE BPD COSTS

BPD imposes an incredible toll on the sufferers, families, and society. Experts believed that around 2-3 percent of the general population had BPD for a long time. Recent findings, however, indicate that this calculation may have underestimated significantly the extent of the problem.

In the following sections, many people with BPD manage to have brilliant careers and live long, fairly successful lives, despite the bleak topics we cover. However, the passage of time typically results in decreased frequency of BPD symptoms, and medication may speed up the process. Don't give up, in other words, because you have many reasons to hope!

Health Costs

Professionals consider BPD as one of the most serious mental illnesses. Approximately 10 percent of people with BPD eventually kill themselves, and much more seriously injure themselves in attempted suicide. Multiple studies carried out from the 1940s to the present have consistently found that people with severe mental illnesses (such as BPD) die young — shockingly, studies show that people with BPD live lives 20 to 25 years shorter than those without mental illness. A lot of factors contribute to such premature deaths. First, people with mental disorders, including BPD, often resort to cigarette smoking as a desperate coping strategy— an obvious risk factor. Also, in addition, people with mental illness typically have more difficulty controlling urges and therefore finding stopping even more challenging than others do. Additionally, researchers find higher rates of obesity and diabetes in BPD sufferers— researchers now consider both of these disorders to be nearly as bad as cigarette smoking in terms of their health risks. Additional risks people with BPD bring with them include elevated heart disease and stroke odds. Unfortunately, some of the drugs used by mental health professionals to treat mental illnesses make matters worse by leading to additional weight gain (and increased risk of heart disease, stroke, and diabetes accompanying it). People with chronic mental illnesses are usually given insufficient basic healthcare due to lack of financial resources.

Accidental death rates and violence-related death are also significantly higher in people with mental illnesses like BPD. Risky, impulsive behaviors can lead to unintentional deaths due to traffic accidents, overdoses of drugs, or sexually transmitted diseases. People with mental illness are also more likely to be homeless because of poor nutrition, lack of health care, poor living conditions, and victimization.

Financial and Career-Related Costs

BPD can exert a disastrous impact on jobs and career opportunities. People with BPD tend to be chronically underemployed — partly because they can begin to idealize new job opportunities, only to become disillusioned and disappointed when jobs don't live up to their inflated expectations. Those with BPD often have trouble understanding who they are, and this often leads them to move from job to job because they don't know where they want to go in life. Eventually, because many people with BPD fail to get along with other people, they frequently lose or quit their jobs because of relationship problems in the workplace.

On the other hand, certain people with BPD are extremely successful in their careers. They may be unusually skillful and gifted. Most of these shockingly accomplished people often respond to their co-workers in negative ways. For example, they can misunderstand co-workers' intentions and respond to the slightest provocation with hypersensitivity and rage. Their successful careers stand in stark contrast to their failed relationships.

The Toll on Family And Friends

Marriage isn't as popular among people with BPD as it is among people that don't have the disorder. And when people with BPD get married, not as many of them choose to have kids compared to the general public. Perhaps surprisingly, their divorce rate does not seem to differ markedly from that among the rest of the population. Family members of BPD people are suffering right along with their loved ones. It is not easy to watch their loved ones cycle through periods of self-harm, suicide attempts, out of control emotions, risky behaviors, and substance abuse. Often partners, parents, and relatives feel helpless. Partners also walk away in frustration and anger from trying to help. In turn, BPD-afflicted families have to contend with the challenges of inadequate treatment programs, discrimination, and stigma. The treatment process is lengthy and expensive, even if families do receive care. Apparently, in addition to its particular victims, BPD casts a wide net of suffering that affects a lot of people.

BPD's Impact on The Healthcare System

BPD costs a lot of money to the worldwide healthcare system, and interestingly, BPD can cost more money when it is not treated than when it is. Some of those costs stem from the issues of personal health that often follow BPD. Such health problems cause people with BPD to go to the doctor more often, and a large number of people with BPD receive their health care in emergency rooms due to chronic underemployment, which is the priciest source of medical care. At least 10 percent of all patients with mental health is diagnosed with BPD. They strongly suspect that this number is poor because a lot of mental health professionals are hesitant to give their patients this diagnosis. This hesitation is a direct response to concerns about stigmatizing patients, as well as the fact that some insurance companies refuse to pay for personality-related services. Besides, BPD accounts for 15 to 20 percent of all mental health hospital patients. Inpatient treatment for mental health continues to be extremely expensive, and costs are rising rapidly. Politicians often see these costs as prohibitive— a view that leads to the underfunding of such services. Because publicly funded programs for mental health treatment are terribly inadequate, some people with BPD end up homeless or in prisons and jails rather than in hospitals or ambulatory settings.

CHAPTER TWO: CAUSES OF BPD; WHO GETS BPD AND WHY?

Not everyone with a horrible experience in childhood ends up with borderline personality disorder (BPD). Many people with BPD report difficult or stressful childhoods, though. Recent studies suggest that combinations of genetic influences are usually present in people who develop BPD, followed by extremely stressful developmental events. Additionally, culture and society create conditions that either promote or inhibit BPD growth. Scientists can not identify a single, direct mechanism leading to the emergence of BPD in a given person. Consider the flu to be a simple illustration. Each time people are exposed to the flu virus, they do not come down with flu. Other factors, such as the genetic makeup of the person, general health, current stress levels, and history (for example, having received a flu shot), make a difference in whether or not a particular person will come down with the flu. Similarly, exposure to one or two risk factors does not cause everybody to have BPD.

Culture Consideration

Culture is identical to the idea of personality. Personality tries to capture a person's essence; culture tries to capture the essence of a society. Culture stands for recurring patterns of behavior, attitudes, convictions, and ways of expressing emotions common to a wide community of people. Culture conveys deep beliefs about how individual members of a given community will live their lives. The manner in which people express emotional distress is also affected by culture. For example, cutting oneself deliberately is a rare and confusing phenomenon in most poor countries. Nevertheless, the act of self-mutilation is a fairly common occurrence in wealthier cultures, particularly among troubled adolescents. Many mental disorders, such as schizophrenia and obsessive-compulsive disorder, arise in most cultures at around the same pace and in similar ways.

Symptoms of BPD occur in different cultures, however, at different rates. The differing social norms across cultures can explain this disparity, at least in part, in the rate of occurrence. The following sections address the following five factors that vary across societies and may have an effect on how often BPD occurs: ibid. Individualism ibid. Adolescence ibid. Entitlement ibid. Family dysfunction ibid. Technology Individualism: Emphasizing me versus we Since the days before the Declaration of Independence, American culture actively encouraged individual freedom. Parents, teachers, and other role models today encourage youth to strive for achievement on their own — to be all they can be. Quality in the U.S. is calculated by how much more you gain or how much better you are at a particular skill than anybody else around you. People are movers in the USA, and in many other modern societies.

People are moving away to improve their own lives or to experience something new. Most modern industrialized countries share the tradition of individual celebrations.

On the other hand, more traditional cultures, like those in the Far East, promote society, family, and interdependence. Many societies prioritize giving the family group respect. People have more structure within their communities in traditional cultures. Families–both nuclear and extended –have mutual support. Unlike more modern cultures, being part of a group, in traditional cultures, is more important than being an individual.

Which has to do with BPD, the focus on the individual versus the group?

Researchers highlighted the alarming scarcity of BPD research across different cultures. While BPD symptoms clearly show up at varying rates across cultures, no one knows the exact BPD incidence around the world. However, a number of researchers have noted that many of the BPD symptoms occur more frequently in cultures that emphasize individual needs, values, and priorities over those of the community at large. Several scientists believe this finding is accompanied by definition, known as self-absorption. Self-absorption refers to a narrow focus on oneself and an increased concern to assess that self. Social scientists have discovered that excessive self-centering substantially increases the risk of a wide range of physical and emotional problems, including eating disorders, anger, alcoholism, substance abuse, self-harm, depression, anxiety, or seeking sensation. A number of psychologists have suggested that excessive self-emphasis creates stress and pressure that leads to these symptoms and other similar ones. A group with strong social ties and an effective system of support will eliminate a lot of that burden. Please understand People with BPD are not blamed for being too self-absorbed. Nobody requires or asks for BPD, and people often don't pursue self-absorption. Modern culture, we believe, is fostering this trait among its people. Self-absorption is, moreover, but one of many contributors to BPD development.

Adolescence and BPD

Adolescence is a relatively modern concept that refers to the period of transition from childhood to adulthood. As a result of the Industrial Revolution, puberty emerged as a way of keeping children out of sweatshops and in school— not such a bad idea. Yet as it has progressed, for many teenagers, puberty has become a turbulent and dangerous time.

Adolescence probably brings with it a lot of free time, which means many opportunities for teens to engage in self-destructive behaviors. To teenagers, pressures keep rising to get more, be more, and be heard. Adolescence is a period when psychological disorders arise, including symptoms of disorders of personality, such as BPD. In the past four or five decades, problems with gangs, crime, drug use, thrill-seeking, eating disorders and risky sexual behavior have grown exponentially among teenagers.

Obviously, we don't assume that puberty itself triggers emotional disorders; after all, many teens develop into adulthood without any evidence of emotional disorders. From a historical perspective, however, BPD symptoms and behaviors have been written about only in the past century or so— which correlate with the rise of puberty as a characteristic of modern culture. There was much less teenage anxiety among teens when kids were busy milking cows and collecting crops. Perhaps if we can give teens more important tasks than text, video gaming, and hanging out at the mall, self-destructive behaviors won't seduce them as easily.

Entitlement: Feeling Too Good

The value of suffering-both physical and emotional-has decreased in recent years. Some hundred years ago, people were admiring others because of their ability to endure suffering. Ancient religious writings, for example, are full of messages which argue in favor of suffering. Many people thought suffering strengthened character and helped people appreciate life's gifts. The message has dramatically changed in modern, industrialized societies. People today resort to drugs to combat the slightest emotional distress, and advertising encourages people to treat their frowns, lines, and splotches just as they do diseases. Yet natural grief has become an uncommon state in need of medical treatment in response to the loss. Sadly, an inability to accept any negative feelings usually increases the susceptibility of a person to get overwhelmed by emotional distress. People who think that feeling good all the time is a fundamental human right will end up feeling entitled to have all their needs met. As a result, they are deeply disappointed when the universe does not appeal to all their needs. Don't get this wrong; of course, everyone likes to feel good. No one definitely is promoting the idea of misery for the sake of suffering. Nonetheless, the ability to withstand anger, delay gratification, and make a full recovery from disappointment are hallmarks of a healthy personality, and people who lack such qualities still fail to remain calm and buoyant with every little mishap that comes along.

Family Instability

Today more children are growing up in single-parent families than ever before, especially in western cultures. While divorce rates have peaked and then gradually decreased over the past ten or twenty years, they remain much higher than in 1950. In fact, fewer people marry today than in the past, and they marry later in life when they do marry. However, large extended families consisting of multiple generations— sisters, aunts, uncles, and grandparents — aren't as usual as they once were. Today, immediate families (for example, mom, dad, and two children) spread all over the world. As a result, the emotional support networks are far less reliable and secure than they once were. Again, it is not known to what extent family dysfunction leads to BPD growth, but social scientists have long recognized that social support acts as a powerful protective force against declining mental and physical health outcomes.

Technology and Its Isolating Effects

Technology has increased productivity, access to information, and the ability to communicate in the form of computers, mobile phones, and the Internet. Everyone loves computers personally— they have helped us to write more and study more easily than ever before. Sometimes we spend days holed up in our offices at a time, banging away on the computer and not talking to other living creatures. But, as we don't want to lose actual, face-to-face contact, we're trying to monitor our isolation to make sure we're not going overboard with cyber communication. Unfortunately, several people are drawn into a new, virtual world that is becoming more thrilling than their actual lives. They spend socializing day after day on Facebook, Twitter, and online gaming pages. They lose contact with the people around them, and in their virtual selves, they become fully absorbed.

Consider how many people choose to relate to others:

Joining a World of Warcraft team rather than a soccer team

Partaking in live webinars rather than meeting friends in a local coffee shop

Making comments on discussion boards rather than communicating face-to-face in social environments

Having conversations via emails and text messages rather than telephoning.

Being a part of anonymous online support groups rather than attending local support group meetings

Cyberstalking friends' profiles rather than getting to know them personally, Of course, some of these ways of "techno-relating" are fun and beneficial.

The Web's social elements appeal to many as they provide simpler, healthier, and faster ways to connect with others. No one really knows how isolation from the overuse of technological ways to relate to others contributes to BPD development or other emotional problems.

Technology can, however, prevent the contact you need to build relationships and trust in people. People with BPD need real relationships, real social support, and real feedback on their behaviour, to get better.

Childhood Challenges and The Increased Risk Of Bpd

Mental health professionals broadly ascribe the theory that mental health in adolescence and adulthood is greatly affected by the events of a childhood. Parents and their way of parenting greatly influence their children's mental and emotional conditions throughout their lives. Those influencing children are other family members, peers, classrooms, communities, acquaintances, and even strangers. Additionally, random events, like hurricanes and house fires, may forever change the lives of young people. However, as important as the impact of childhood is on humans, bear in mind that children are quite resilient. In drawing connections between childhood problems and disorders in adulthood, many mental health professionals have allowed their opinions to run before data. BPD development, as research has shown, involves much more than mere poor parenting or even traumatic events. Many children experience significant traumas as well as neglected parents, yet they manage to lead healthy emotional lives. A biological vulnerability typically has at least one part to play in BPD development. Nonetheless, stressful childhoods do increase the risks of developing BPD. The three major factors that can negatively affect childhood and, as a result, can increase the risk for BPD in some situations are neglect and trauma, parenting styles, and early separation and loss. BPD has no specific cause. In order to increase the likelihood of BPD, most of the issues described in the following sections must have occurred in extreme forms and/or for a very long period of time. Even then, for BPD to emerge, they generally require some interaction with biological and cultural factors.

Problematic Parenting

Most of what mental health professionals learn about people's parents who have BPD comes from reports from people who have BPD. But when people suffer great distress, they tend to focus on negative events and remember them far more than positive ones. Once they feel better, they have a somewhat more optimistic quality in their descriptions of certain things. As a consequence, researchers are constantly arguing over how much weight to give studies based on such memories. Unfortunately, far fewer studies at a given point in time look objectively at parenting styles and then follow the outcomes in terms of how children function in adulthood. Current professional views on parenting and its true long-term effects therefore remain quite grim. At the same time, there has been a strong degree of agreement among mental health professionals that certain parenting strategies affect children. The following sections take a look at some problematic parenting styles.

Emotional Invalidation

Psychologist Marsha Linehan supports the idea that emotional illness plays a critical role in promoting BPD growth. Emotional disability applies to a variety of ways parents undermine, demean, underestimate, and disqualify emotional experiences of children. Parents who emotionally vitiate their children send their children a wide variety of messages, which ultimately teach them to distrust or disbelieve their own emotional reactions. In the following list, we explore some of the more common messages that parents use to invalidate the emotions of their children and describe how these messages affect the feelings of the children:

That isn't how you should feel: Parents send messages like this one when their children are upset or hurt. Parents may feel uncomfortable with the distress of their children and, by using this message, try to squelch that. Parents may think they help their children calm down, but the message's net effect is to cause shame and to invalidate the feelings of the children.

What are you shedding tears for: Most people don't like hearing others cry. In fact, some parents have a very low tolerance to deal with the extremely grating noise that is generated by crying and wailing. Unfortunately, kids can't really answer this question because they feel overwhelmed and often just don't know the answer. Parents suggest that anxiety and sorrow are not suitable feelings with this message.

You exaggerate a lot: This message basically tells kids they are fundamentally misinterpreting reality. Consequently, children learn to distrust their perceptions. This argument seeks to suppress feelings instead of teaching children how to control them.

That's just not valid: Children sometimes come to parents with opinions on relationships, school, or even politics. Instead of encouraging independent thinking, parents lead kids to distrust their own viewpoints and rely on superior knowledge from their parents instead. This argument is likewise quite a stopper for conversation.

You are the same as your dad (brother, uncle, aunt, or whomever): The message invalidates children's very identities. Comparisons with other family members usually aren't particularly flattering. Using this message hampers the development of children and their desire to trust in their own abilities.

I'm sure you'd like to be more like your sister (cousin, brother, aunt or whomever): This message tells children they're not good enough and their parents are disappointed about who they are. This message erodes the identities of children, once again.

You should grow up: Children are busy, distracting, and, well, just kids by definition. Parents who can't bear anger typically put their children down for childlike boisterous behavior. Not only does this message not alter the attitudes of children, but it also makes them feel bad for acting like children.

Tell me a good thing that's happened: Many parents say this when their children report a troubling or sad incident. These parents believe that redirecting the child to focus on more pleasant events, rather than validating the sadness, will help them learn to feel better. Rather, that approach teaches children to suppress their true emotions.

You are selfish: In truth, the majority of children are a bit selfish. They have not yet learned to fully appreciate other people's needs, expectations, and opinions or to align those needs with their own. Alas, this message does not motivate them to become less selfish. Instead, it invalidates children because they are true to their existence.

You're so much too young to do something like this: You could (hurt yourself, get into trouble, get lost, or whatever). Always ask me before you do anything at all! Some parents use messages such as this one because of their own insecurity and wish to protect their children. Sadly this approach suppresses the interest, freedom, inspiration, confidence, and competence of children. Growing up in a family where the world is dominated by mental illness can be very hurtful for children. Children either learn to withdraw passively to prevent such messages, or to exhibit extreme emotions and actions in order to gain respect and attention.

Dysfunctional and Disorganized Families

Dysfunction occurs when there is high marital discord and conflict among parents. Many parents communicate this tension freely in the form of constant loud fights that fill children with anxiety and even fear that one or both parents can abandon them. Some spouses, behind closed doors, show these marital problems. The parents can cover up in these cases and refuse to discuss their disagreements. While this strategy may sound less traumatic to kids, most experts agree that sweeping problems under the rug make them just grow out of control. Children take on the subtle signs of frustration, and when parents don't settle their disputes freely with each other, their kids fail to learn the skills necessary to resolve their own conflicts. Dysfunction often occurs when parents put their children into conflicting roles and expectations.

Many parents feel practically incapable of parenting and imposing undue expectations on their older children— making them virtually parents of the younger children. Other parents take the opposite approach and treat their children as incompetent — making them seem like infants in essence. Many homes are riddled with disorganized chaos, something that is often hard to understand and handle for children. Such chaos comes in a wide variety of forms, including:

Financial woes, unpaid bills, and bill collectors

Frequent job changes

Constant moves from one neighborhood to another

Conflicts that cause various household members to move in and out

Substance abuse

Incarceration

Neighborhood crime

Disability, serious illness, or severe emotional disorders in one or more of the parents

Such kinds of noisy atmospheres confuse children and make it very difficult to grasp the feelings of their own and of other people. The chaotic disorder often interferes with the developmentally important process of learning how to manage or regulate emotions.

Abuse and Trauma

Multiple studies have shown that people with BPD in their childhood have a high rate of abuse— caused either by their parents or by someone else, namely a friend, a bully, or a stranger. Many experts believe that BPD is, in fact, a complex type of post-traumatic stress disorder (also called PTSD) because of such evidence. Many researchers now, however, maintain that BPD is not a type of PTSD, while trauma definitely increases the risk of developing BPD. One reason researchers believe that BPD is separate from PTSD is that BPD can and does develop in people whose childhoods do not show clear signs of trauma. Biological vulnerabilities combine with other difficulties, such as emotionally disabling experiences or chaotic childhoods, and lead to BPD in some people.

Many individuals, on the other hand, go through traumatic events and don't develop BPD or even PTSD. Many of the people who show great resilience to trauma are likely to do so because of their genetic makeup, which helps them to survive challenges that many others cannot. Other factors, such as highly supportive families, the presence of a particularly involved caring adult, or psychotherapy, can also serve as a protective function for some individuals who experience traumatic events.

In addition, the kind of trauma experienced by children makes a difference in whether they develop BPD or other emotional disorders later in life. The trauma suffered by a trusted member of the family seems to have a greater impact than trauma caused by an outsider.

Sexual molestation, which has usually been going on for years has a greater impact than a single molestation case. Incest is usually more likely to increase the risk of BPD and other emotional disorders than molestation by a stranger. Nevertheless, keep in mind that any incident involving child abuse or trauma causes harm. However, in the absence of genetic instability or other risk factors, many children eventually succeed in overcoming some of the harmful effects.

Separation and Loss

Over extended periods of time, sudden losses and separation from one or more parents contribute to increased risk of BPD. These losses can be quite upsetting because they interfere with the formation of normal bonding between children and parents. Kids who lose parents often get more nervous and partially depressed as they think about who's going to take care of them. Nevertheless, like the case of trauma and abuse, for the most part, some children lose a parent and surmount the consequences of the loss. These recoveries are more likely when these children have an underlying biological resilience and don't have the other risk factors of BPD.

Genetics and Biology

BPD indicates in the Family Tree Studies that BPD can as well be hereditary. When one person has BPD, the probability that a close relative also has BPD is about ten times greater. Yet bear in mind that there are many people living together in the same family or having similar childhoods. But childhood can be responsible for the higher BPD levels in the same family, rather than genetics. You might wonder at this point how to find out what's in the genes, and what's coming from the background.

Personality Traits, Genes, And BPD

Since BPD is a personality disorder, you can wonder what kinds of traits or behaviors are related to BPD? So, what are the personality traits exactly? Personality traits are ways of thinking, feeling, and behaving that remain pretty much the same throughout your life through different situations. These are the characteristics of who you actually are. When someone says, "He loves to socialize with others" or "He's an introvert," they really talk about traits of personality.

Genes of impulsivity and of dopamine

One BPD-related personality trait is impulsivity, the propensity to behave quickly, on the spur of the moment, without thinking things through. You may have found that if you have BPD, you appear to be on the impulsive side. You may be making very quick decisions without considering what might happen as a consequence. For example, you might choose to go home with someone you've just met, without considering the fact that you might get hurt. Or, you might choose an impulse to gorge on food or use drugs without considering all the negative consequences.

Impulsivity is a BPD characteristic that can cause you trouble and anxiety. In fact, BPD people tend to be more impulsive than BPD-free people and people with other personality disorders. Those with BPD also have higher rates of other personality traits similar to impulsiveness, such as looking for novelty (the tendency to look for interesting or novel situations). Furthermore, impulsiveness is associated with attempted suicide in people with BPD. The higher your impulsiveness is, the more likely you have tried suicide in the past. Findings from some studies have suggested that people with some form of the DRD4 gene may have lower dopamine production and may have impulsivity-related traits, such as searching for novelty. Dopamine is a drug that affects the mood in your brain, your sense of pleasure and the regulation of body movement. Obviously, this dopamine gene doesn't describe all impulsive behavior events, and the results have been mixed up till now.

Negative thoughts and serotonin genes.

Another range of BPD-related personality traits includes sensitivity to negative emotions. One of these traits is called neuroticism, which is the propensity to feel negative emotions. If you have a high level of neuroticism, you're definitely experiencing a lot of negative emotions daily. This is one of BPD's strengths, of course, so if you have BPD, you're definitely no stranger to negative emotions. Sometimes we all experience negative feelings, and all of us have a certain degree of neuroticism. It is actually that some are more neurotic than others. Evidence tells us that people with BPD appear to get higher scores on neuroticism tests than people without BPD. Those with BPD also score higher on tests of neuroticism-related personality traits, such as harm avoidance (the inclination to avoid dangerous or potentially harmful activities) and anxiety. Now, this is probably not surprising at all. By now, you know BPD people are very emotional. And there is nothing wrong with going through intense, negative emotions. What's most important is what you do with those emotions. Several researchers have been looking into neuroticism to see what genes are correlated with this characteristic of personality. Some people think that the serotonin, which is secreted by the brain may be associated with negative emotions, depression, anxiety, and neuroticism. Serotonin is a neurotransmitter, which regulates, among other things, mood, appetite, temperature, sexual activity, sleep, and aggression. Several studies have shown that people who score high in neuroticism are likely to have some type of a gene that is linked to low serotonin activity levels (compared to people who are not neurotic or do not have that form of the gene). So, having some form of this gene may make it more likely that individuals will have low serotonin production and higher negative emotions (neuroticism). In effect, if you have high levels of negative emotions, you may have greater chance of developing BPD.

BORDERLINE PERSONALITY DISORDER AND THE BRAIN

If you have BPD, you may have wondered if your brain is somehow different from those of people without BPD. You may have found that you are responding to things differently than other people around you do. You may think differently, feel more intense emotions, or have more trouble stopping you from engaging in impulsive actions. If so, you might have wondered if you're simply having a different type of brain than others do. This isn't as easy as that, as it turns out. The brain is very complex, with many different structures and processes communicating with each other in ways that scientists are just beginning to understand. There might have been variations in your brain from birth or even before birth, or overtime they might have grown. Several factors can affect the functioning of the brain and even the size of certain brain areas. Brain variations between people with BPD and those without BPD may be caused by genes; exposure to adverse conditions or substances during gestation (stressful events, drugs, medication, or alcohol usage); stressful events during infancy, adolescence, or later; use of alcohol; use of drugs; or any number of other things that affect the brain. Below we'll go through some of the areas of the brain that might be involved in BPD. These are the limbic system, the prefrontal cortex, and the hypothalamic-pituitary-adrenal axis.

THE LIMBIC SYSTEM AND THE PREFRONTAL CORTEX

The limbic system is a region of your brain which has to do with, among other things, feelings, memory, and pleasure. Some of the limbic system's brain structures include the amygdala and hippocampus. The amygdala is essentially the brain's emotional centre. Your amygdala becomes responsive when you encounter an emotional event and becomes engaged. Conversely, the hippocampus is involved in learning and memory. BPD is an emotional disorder, as explained. If you have BPD, you are likely to experience intense emotions that sometimes change quite rapidly and stick around for an agonizingly long time at other times. You may also have trouble getting down once you are feeling a strong emotion. Therefore, it's probably not surprising that researchers have found variations in the amygdala of BPD people and BPD-free people. The research shows that people with BPD have smaller amygdala compared to those who do not have BPD, and some areas of their amygdala are more reactive to emotional stimulation. For example, one study monitored how the amygdala behaved when research people looked at faces with different types of emotional expressions (such as sorrow, or anger). Those with BPD were more triggered in their left amygdala. Research has also demonstrated that people with BPD tend to have a smaller hippocampus than those without BPD. It is interesting to note that people with post-traumatic stress disorder (PTSD) also tend to have a smaller hippocampus but that both the hippocampus and the amygdala are smaller only among people with BPD. Another area of the brain that seems to be associated with BPD is the prefrontal cortex, a small but very complex area of the brain that has many different functions involved.

There's some suggestion that prefrontal cortex activity affects some of the limbic system activity (including the amygdala). Essentially, activity in the prefrontal cortex seems to be able to keep the activity in check in this brain's emotional core. Interestingly, some of the BPD research has found that people with BPD report reduced activation in certain prefrontal cortex areas (such as the anterior cingulate cortex, among other regions) when subjected to traumatic memories). When people with BPD have low levels of prefrontal cortex activity, then the prefrontal cortex may not be sufficiently involved in some ways to curb amygdala function. As a result, their emotions can spin out of control when they experience a stressful event.

THE HYPOTHALAMIC-PITUITARY-ADRENAL AXIS

Another area of the brain relating to BPD is the hypothalamic-pituitary-adrenal axis or the HPA axis. Two of the brain structures within the HPA axis are the pituitary gland and the hypothalamus. Both of these areas affect your body's response to stress, and higher activity in the HPA axis results in higher concentrations of a stress hormone called cortisol in your system. When researchers study the axis of HPA, they often get people to give samples of saliva to see how much cortisol is in their systems. This is an indirect indicator of how involved an aspect of your HPA is. Generally speaking, the more active this is, the more cortisol is in your system. So an overly active (or hyperactive) HPA axis means you've got a hyperactive response to biological stress. If you have BPD, you might have found that sometimes you're pushed over the edge by stressors that seem insignificant to others. You may go through times where you feel extremely stressed and get upset at even the smallest things, such as your computer not functioning properly, forgetting to put out the garbage before the garbage truck arrives, losing your keys, receiving complaints from your boss at work, spilling your coffee or any of the other daily problems and stresses that we all encounter on a regular basis You may find that, in other words, you sometimes have an excessive response to stress. Some research on the HPA axis has found that people with BPD demonstrate exaggerated cortisol responses compared to those who do not have BPD. Other studies have found that hyperactivity in the HPA axis may predispose people to suicide attempts. The important thing to know is that stressful and traumatic experiences in life will increase your chances of excessive cortisol response and hyperactivity in the HPA axis. It does make sense, doesn't it? If you're seriously hurt or traumatized, your body may say, "Oh, it's time to prepare my system just in case this happens again." The reaction to cortisol is part of your body's stress response. So, the body may start becoming too sensitive for its own good by experiencing very stressful events. You may feel extremely anxious about even relatively minor stuff (like spilling your coffee), as described above. From time to time, this kind of reaction happens to all of us— we can think of many occasions when we get more stressed out than we expected when driving, after spilling something, or when a printer or photocopier is not working properly. But if you have BPD, this could happen to you even more or more often than not. And this may be due, in part, to the biological effects of previous stressful life experiences.

CHAPTER THREE: TAKING NOTE OF THE MAJOR SYMPTOMS

IMPULSIVE BEHAVIOR

Impulsivity includes two issues with sensitive behavior. First, People who act impulsively tend to overlook the future, especially the negative consequences that are likely to result from their current behaviors. Second, impulsive people don't process information fully until they act. They don't think, in other words, before acting. Those with BPD have trouble controlling their urges, or they have urgent desires and needs. They are craving excitement and drama, and they want it now — hence the term sensation seekers. They feel driven to fill the deep well of emptiness they feel inside, but they only increase their feelings of hollowness with every impulsive behavior. The more they try to fulfill their insatiable fears, the more their anxieties intensify. They typically report feeling momentarily better after they engage in an impulsive act. But those feelings of happiness are rapidly replaced by massive remorse, fear, and self-loathing.

Individuals with BPD find several different ways to satisfy their sensation-seeking desires. Here are some of the more common habits people with BPD rely on to meet their urges:

Some expenditure: impulsive expenditure is not about walking by a fun box in the grocery store and buying it on impulses. Every now and then, most people buy something on impulse. However, in contrast, problematic, impulsive spending involves buying binges out of control. Many people with BPD try to fill a gap by purchasing excessive amounts of absolutely unnecessary things. Some impulsive spenders pile debt in a landfill like a mountain of trash. People who spend impulsively can go on extravagant holidays, spend too much on luxuries, and fill wardrobes with clothes they rarely even wear — all to fill the emptiness within.

Gambling: Gambling in most developed countries is a rapidly growing problem. Those who go to a casino regularly and spend a set amount of money don't count as impulsive players. Many people know winning chances are with the casino, not the gambler. However, those odds are ignored by some people with BPD and gamble with abandon. They sometimes take out second-hand mortgages to fuel their habits. They may even succumb to forgery, embezzlement, and fraud in order to raise the money we need to keep playing. In most situations, as with impulsive buying, the reason is to fill a rush of excitement with the loneliness they feel inside, but it never succeeds — at least not in the long term.

Binge eating: BPD people sometimes try to regulate their emotions by over-eating and fill their feelings of emptiness. They binge on a whole box of cookies, and ice cream carton, or a giant potato chip bag. They eat such large amounts that they often vomit, or at least feel an acute discomfort, rather than feel satisfied.

Shoplifting: often, you read about a movie star or other famous, wealthy person who gets caught shoplifting from time to time. You're likely wondering why people with tons of money risk jail time for something they can afford to buy quickly. The answer lies in the excitement they require. Individuals with BPD who are impulsive shoplifters fill the void of their lives with the excitement that comes with shoplifting — and perhaps even terror. Sometimes relatively worthless items are stolen just to give them away. Keep in mind that impulsive shoplifters are not thieves due to the dire economic conditions.

Reckless driving: Reckless drivers ignore all of their behavior's potential consequences. To add excitement and a sense of danger to their lives, they initiate reckless behavior. Individuals with BPD who demonstrate this risky behavior do incredibly dangerous things on the road— shooting through stoplights, changing lanes without signaling to other drivers, driving well beyond the limit, and unlawfully performing hair-raising U-turns. If you're curious if impulsive, reckless drivers end up in more collisions than others, studies show the answer is yes.

Reckless sex: Sex is thrilling for many people Individuals with BPD who display impulsive behaviors frequently try to increase their excitation by looking for one new partner after another. Even though their current partner fears abandonment, they often have affairs and engage in risky, unprotected sexual activities. They may be seduced by sadomasochistic sex, group sex, swapping of partners, or exhibitionism. For people who follow their sexual impulses, sex with someone new may be an effort to get the affirmation they were not getting as adolescents. And, they may use sex to try and fill their lives with the loneliness they feel. Such impulsive sexual behavior certainly greatly increases the risk of sexually transmitted diseases, unwanted pregnancies, and sometimes even abuse.

Abuse of substances: substance abuse is one of the most common forms of impulsiveness that people engage in, whether or not they have BPD. Additionally, the intake of many drugs (such as alcohol, marijuana, cocaine, or ecstasy) induces more failure of control and activates further impulsive behaviors of other types. Many people who have BPD misuse drugs to try to regulate their feelings out of control. Some do so because they want to fill their endless void for the rush or the big.

Unfortunately, the risk of suicide in people with BPD who are already at high risk of self-induced death increases with substance abuse. Impulsivity partially explains why most people with BPD do not survive without the condition as long as people can. BPD all too often cuts life short, whether due to suicide, car crashes, substance abuse, or even unhealthy lifestyles.

SUICIDAL OR SELF-HARMING BEHAVIOR

Self-harm is a more severe impulsive BPD symptom than the actions identified in the section above. Most people assume acts of self-injury or mutilation are suicide attempts; however, a desire to die is typically not the motivation that causes somebody to cause self-harm.

Individuals with BPD are at an alarmingly high risk of committing suicide ultimately. The vulnerability frightens the people who care for them and scares the mental health care professionals who help them. These suicidal acts are among the most severe and complex of impulsive behaviors that affect people with BPD at times. People who live through attempted suicide usually report having felt unbearable emotional pain before the attempt. Their options and their lives felt helpless and hopeless. They saw no potential for a better future, and the idea of oblivion left them with no alternative choice. Suicide attempts are occasionally desperate calls for help. Sadly support comes too late for people who succeed in suicide. Suicide attempts for other people seem to involve a need to get back to people in their lives who have wronged them, abandoned them, or hurt them. In such cases, people with suicidal urges seem to believe that after their death, they will be able to watch their foes feel guilt and remorse.

Types of Self-Harming Acts

People with BPD perform a surprisingly diverse variety of acts, all intended to inflict pain or harm on themselves, including the following: Cutting: people who use this self-harming technique most often cut their hands, legs, and stomach. Many cutters are trying to hide their injuries whilst others are trying to show them. They use different tools, such as razor blades, scissors, clips on paper, pins, needles, knives, and broken glass. Sometimes, people even scratch their own fingernails severely.

Burning: cigarettes, lighters, and matches are often used by people with BPD to burn themselves. Each burning act typically involves only a small area of the body; however, many scars may spread over time.

Blunt force trauma: This category of self-harm includes pounding the fist against walls, punching oneself, banging the head into something hard, and using a hammer or other tool to inflict pain on their own body. Blunt force trauma also leads to bruises, cuts, wounds, and, in rare cases, broken bones.

Removing the skin and pulling the hair: removing cuticles and scabs, pulling the hair out, and pinching the skin until it bleeds. Sometimes these signs often accompany various other mental conditions and may be linked to obsessive-compulsive disorder.

Intentional accidents: at first, actions in this self-harm group may seem unintended. Many people with BPD deliberately avoid taking reasonable precautions, however. Many may have workplace or home injuries that they could easily avoid by being more vigilant or using basic safety equipment or clothing. They can fall off ladders which they set up on the unstable ground or burn themselves while using broken sticks to rearrange logs in a fireplace, as a result of not being careful.

While you may wonder why some people want to hurt themselves, people with BPD and therapists who treat them have developed a lot of hypotheses about the reasons behind these disturbing and extremely painful behaviors.

Such reasons include the following:

To get attention: Most experts do not agree that this motive plays a significant role in the rationale behind most self-harming actions because most people who are self-harming try to hide from others what they have done. However, people with BPD sometimes lack the skills they need to get adequate nurturing and support from others. Then they feel compelled to harm themselves as a way of seeking aid. Ultimately, these attention-seeking deeds may give rise to the interest and care of people with BPD need, but they are desperate ways to achieve this goal.

To escape from emotional pain: many experts believe that people with BPD are involved in self-harm as a means of dealing with intense internal or emotional distress. Physical pain pales in comparison to what they feel internally, but it does, at least temporarily, draw attention away from their overwhelming emotions.

To feel better: your brain releases natural pain killers called endorphins when you are injured. Such endorphins will ease the return to a less distressing emotional state. Therefore, physical pain can, surprisingly, potentially help some people control their emotions. Many people find appeal in eating hot chili peppers for a far less extreme example of the positive effects of endorphins, as eating them allows their bodies to release endorphins. So even people who don't suffer from severe emotional disorders can understand the appeal of getting a rush of endorphins at some level.

Feeling anything but numbness and emptiness: Some people with BPD report feeling unreal and out of touch with the world around them. To punish themselves: while mental health professionals don't know how often this incentive leads people with BPD to self-harming activities, some people do say that they feel they deserve to be punished and harmed. The self-harm can be a way for people to punish themselves in these situations.

To get back to someone: some people with BPD are unable to express their anger adequately and hurt to make others feel guilty of something they have said or done.

Re-enacting their own abuse: Most people with BPD experience childhood abuse. Children often believe they deserve the abuse they receive, and as adults, they sometimes continue on their own pattern of abuse.

Such theories reflect fascinating motives. Nevertheless, in people with BPD, experts do not have enough evidence to establish which reasons better account for self-harm. The reasons most likely vary for each individual. While you may find it fascinating to study the reasons behind self-harming behaviors, people with BPD who hurt themselves may not see their insight helpful. In other words, insight into why people hurt themselves is not always sufficient to help them stop problems.

IDENTITY AND BPD

Identity is a theory or concept that somebody creates to synthesize information and self-knowledge. In other words, your personal Identity is your own attempt to capture the core elements that make you who you are. Identity evolves over time, as it takes on different areas of focus. A 3-month-old baby, for example, has no sense of gender, but when that baby is 14, she actually thinks a lot about the importance of gender. Children usually don't have much of a career identification in grade school, but in young adulthood, this critical area takes on great significance. On the other hand, personality describes broad character traits that other people can see. By essence, Identity is more personal than personality. In other words, Identity includes judgments of importance that people make about themselves, not opinions that others make about themselves. For example, wealth has little or nothing directly to do with personality; however, people often attach much of their self-worth and personalities to their money accumulation— or lack thereof. Individuals can, therefore, have outgoing personalities and be rich or poor. Their wealth does not have a clear automatic impact on their personalities. Many rich people, for example, believe like their wealth has little to do with who they are as humans. On the other hand, some wealthy people feel as if their worlds are wrapped around their belongings— who they are and what they value.

Identity can be healthy or unhealthy, as can personality. Healthy identities are built on strong, diverse ideals. They're not centering on a single person element. A healthy identity, for example, can encompass multiple sources of self-worth. By comparison, an unhealthy identity has a limited scope and typically derives meaning from just a few components. People with BPD have identities that are different from those of others. Their identities show less consistency and less clarity. Additionally, individuals with BPD frequently overreact to subtle threats to their fragile Identity.

Waffling identities

Even though everyone often behaves inconsistently, people with BPD experience immense variations in behaviors, beliefs, and feelings. The difference between a person without BPD's identities and a person with BPD are much like the difference between a well-edited film about someone's life and an unorganized box jammed with photos from that same life. Here are a few different examples:

A woman without BPD respects integrity, and as a result, she has a stable, coherent sense of fundamental honesty. Therefore, she's very honest with people 99 percent of the time. She's somebody who everybody knows they can truly count on. Meanwhile, she thanks the host for cooking at a friend's house for dinner, although she does not like the food at all. She preserves her true personality and recognizes the fact that certain situations involve lies of a minor nature. The coherent film about her life retains the underlying concept of authenticity.

Sometimes a woman with BPD thinks she's an honest person and is honest in general. She feels a rush of self-loathing and disgust for her dishonest behavior, though, when lying to her friend about her cooking. This situation could lead her to get upset with her friend for "asking" her to tell a lie. In the face of a slight indiscretion, she cannot hang on to her fundamental image of being honest. In a way, with every photo taken out of the box of her life, her sense of who she is, shifts.

A BPD man can find himself extremely just and committed to his family. He often has affairs, however, and loses his temper when his children struggle in the slightest way to meet his standards. He briefly feels horrible about himself after he flips into these obnoxious episodes. Within hours or days, however, he quickly regains his self-image of being just and devoted. His impression of himself dramatically changes, as each picture is taken from the box. Most people with BPD, without a reliable, secure sense of their own identities, try to adopt whatever Identity they think their current partners or friends want them to have. They believe that doing so can make them attractive to their potential partners or friends, because they may appear as the very personification of the dreams of their friends. The intrinsic ambiguity in their personal identities, however, makes it impossible to preserve the facades.

Responding to Identity Concerns

When people with BPD have significant concerns about their Identity and self-worth, one of two situations is likely to occur: either they desperately try to hold on to their fragile sense of self-worth by striking out in rage or their Identity and self-worth collapses, and they drop into a cycle of despair.

CHAPTER FOUR: MAKING THE CHOICE TO CHANGE

Borderline personality disorder (BPD) is a wide cluster of symptoms. Treatment is challenging because of the range of problems people with BPD experience. Some people with BPD, for example, have trouble with substance abuse, difficulty in keeping a job, stormy relationships, or serious mood issues. Some feel empty inside, think about being lost, or try to hurt themselves physically. It can be incredibly difficult to address even one of these issues, so imagine how hard a mixture of them can be to handle. While treatment for BPD takes a while and may at first seem daunting, it usually helps significantly over time. Not surprisingly, the wide range of treatments available makes it challenging for individuals who have BPD or those people who care for them to choose the right treatment. You can choose from one hour a week of individual psychotherapy, day treatment (known as partial hospitalization), full-time hospitalization, or group therapy if you have BPD.

EXPLORING BPD TREATMENT SETTINGS

The BPD diagnosis can be used in a variety of settings. Each of these settings— whether it's working one-on-one with a therapist, engaging in group therapy, or spending time in a hospital— has certain pluses and minus.

Working with a therapist individually

Many mental health professionals work separately and provide individual services, one at a time. They usually see each patient, either once or twice a week, for fifty minutes. Individual counseling once or twice a week may not suffice for people with BPD, especially during times of great turmoil. Yet, with the aid of individual psychotherapy, many people with BPD do get better.

Giving group psychotherapy a chance

Group psychotherapy has been around for a long time, but many people shy away from this form of therapy out of fear of entrusting other people with personal information, particularly those they don't know. Often, they avoid talking in front of a group, or those other members of the group would condemn them. Group therapy, though, can be a very useful part of treating BPD. Group environments provide an excellent way to teach essential competencies and provide knowledge about BPD management. Group therapy is also somewhat more cost-effective than individual therapy because the participants share the costs. Therefore, it can be very encouraging to see that you're not the only one who is struggling the way you are. You may want to continue your care with individual therapy if you find the idea of group therapy too overwhelming. They strongly suggest, however, that you express your group therapy issues with your therapist so that the two of you can overcome those worries.

Spend More Time in Care

Partial Hospitalization: Many local hospitals provide BPD treatment programs in a type known as partial hospitalization. Partial hospitalization programs generally include group therapy, individual therapy, medication, and adjunctive treatment, such as art therapy, physical therapy, and occupational therapy. While researchers have not yet examined such adjunctive therapies in relation to BPD care, time spent on these interventions can be of some benefit to many people, regardless of their condition. For example, a good therapist can use that opportunity to show the patient how to use some practical interpersonal conflict-management skills when a conflict arises in a therapeutic therapy session.

Combining and Changing Therapies

About half of people seeking BPD care receive treatment in more than one type of environment, either concurrently or one after another. You may thus start with individual therapy and then add group therapy later. In addition to your individual and group therapy, you may even be needing partial hospitalization for a few weeks. You may also go to an inpatient setting, but you probably won't stay for long or more than once or twice in that setting. You and your primary individual therapist will work together to determine, at any given time, which therapies are best for you.

Researching the treatment methods that work for BPD

You can find a kaleidoscope of different types of psychotherapy if you take a few minutes to call about different therapists or clinics or search the Internet. Jungian therapy, primal scream therapy, psychoanalysis (in different forms), cognitive therapy, cognitive behavioral therapy, humanistic therapy, Rogerian therapy, haiku therapy, Hakomi therapy, and so on and so forth.

Are you still confused? Okay, don't get overwhelmed. The choice of which treatment to choose can be made a little easier. In fact, only a handful of psychotherapies have shown considerable promise for BPD treatment. You certainly don't want to search for BPD treatment that isn't explicitly designed to handle this condition. Preliminary evidence indicates that non-specific treatment may slow down or delay the natural healing that takes place over time. Research supports BPD recovery approaches such as:

Dialectical behavior therapy (DBT)

Mentalization-based therapy (MBT)

Transference-focused psychotherapy (TFP)

Cognitive therapy

Schema therapy

Medication

Choosing a Mental Health Professional

If you have BPD, you need support from others- usually trained professionals in mental health. Some treatments involve a team of professionals working together, and others involve just one therapist working with you on an individual basis. When you're looking for a mental health professional, you need to ask about the experience and knowledge of BPD treatment specifically. You want somebody who's got experience. If the first person you meet is not confident handling BPD, don't get discouraged. Not everyone is, but you'll probably find someone who's if you call around. When you're in touch with a mental health professional, you need to ask a variety of questions to that professional, including the following:

Where and how often are you available? Tell the provider how easily you can schedule an appointment. Sadly, the providers are so overwhelmed in some areas of the country that they have waiting lists. Others may have a small number of available appointment times. Ask about the hours of the provider— especially if you need weekend or evening hours. BPD treatment includes regularly scheduled meetings, so make sure you set up a weekly meeting time that works for you and the provider alike.

Do you offer emergency after-hours and coverage? Part of the BPD treatment requires dangerous or self-harming behavior. Ask the therapist what emergency arrangements she makes. The practices of therapists range from being on call 24/7 with help when the therapist is out of town to not be available after hours for any reason (in which case the therapist usually gives patients directions to contact 911 or to go to an emergency room in case of an emergency). To date, no research studies have specifically looked at how the therapist's availability improves or hinders BPD care. All strategies have justifiable reasons behind them. What is crucial is that your therapist will set out the policies and procedures in advance, and you will feel comfortable with these.

What fees are you going to charge? Ask the provider what session fees she charges? If your care involves multiple sessions per week, are the individual and group counseling costs different or equal? Does your therapist take your insurance? Many physicians do not accept all plans for insurance, and others do not accept any plans for insurance. In addition, there are insurance plans which do not include mental health. It is advised to check with your insurance plan, as well as the therapist. Often providers may force insurance companies to pay more than their normal rebate when the procedure is a legitimate BPD treatment.

Beginning Treatment

When you decide to start BPD treatment, what are you supposed to do next? Next, you have to expect quite a few questions to answer. These are essential questions that are designed to help your therapist learn about you and your problems. Be prepared to answer questions about the following issues and concerns:

Symptoms:

Symptoms include frustration, rage, depression, anxiety, impulsive behavior, misuse of drugs, self-harming behaviors, suicidal thoughts or acts, difficulties with relationships, etc. Your doctor will ask you questions about all of your symptoms— when did they begin? How are they conflicting with what you want to be doing? How often are they? Which kinds of situations are making them worse? How depressed are you feeling over them?

Physical health issues:

Without a doubt, the doctor will ask you questions about your overall physical wellbeing— How is your sleep? How is your appetite? Were you feeling some physical pain? Did you ever have serious injuries, surgeries, or illnesses? Did you have a recent physical exam? Do you take prescription drugs at all? Do you take medicinal products or supplements over the counter?

History:

Several factors contribute to the development of BPD, including childhood conditions, and your therapist will ask you about your history — have you ever been abused? Ever suffered any kind of trauma? Have you ever been taken into hospital? Have you ever considered suicide or attempted it? Did you take medicine, or have you been treated for any emotional problems before? What is your history of education? What is the history of your work? What is the past of your relationships?

Family:

Because genetics play a role in BPD development, your provider will ask you about your family— Does anybody in your family have any kind of emotional problems? Have any of your family taken mental problems treatment or psychotherapy?

Finances:

Some people express discomfort when discussing financial issues, but your therapist needs to know some basics — are you covered by insurance? Can you afford to take treatment? Is finances a source of stress for your family or for you?

Evaluating the Treatment

A key symptom of BPD involves having relationship problems. Another explanation for this challenge is that people with BPD are easily misinterpreting the context of what others tell them. So if you feel criticized, unsupported, or angered at any time by the words or actions of your therapist, you need to check your concerns. Try not to lash out or walk out, but try to determine what led to your response. Let yourself be open to what your therapist says. Upon having spent half a dozen or so sessions and having checked out any questions you might have, you would usually feel quite comfortable sharing and talking with your therapist about just about anything. You should know you are listening to your therapist, and he/she trusts you as a person. The majority of therapists exhibit reasonable warmth, empathy, and concern.

Giving Therapy Some Time

Psychotherapy for BPD takes a bit of time. Some programs can take as long as three years, such as schema therapy, but the results might be worth the wait. Some systems tend to be much shorter. Nonetheless, before you begin to feel significant progress, you should expect treatment to take at least several months. Most BPD patients remain in treatment for several years. You should reasonably expect to reduce and control the impulses to commit self-harm or suicide within six months to a year of treatment. Other goals, such as improved life satisfaction, reduced impulsiveness, and better relationships, are likely to take much longer. Have some patience. When you give enough time and effort to treatment, you're likely to get better.

Breaking Through Barriers to Changing

People with BPD, fear changes like so many others. They fear it will be complicated, maybe humiliating, and maybe even impossible to get support for their problems. So, they ask themselves why take a chance in the first place if the treatment may not be successful? For many people, it seems better not to try anything at all than to try and fail. Blaming and procrastination, along with anxiety, often pose obstacles to change. Searching for villains or victims fetters people on the spot, unable to move on. Ignoring the signs or discontinuing therapy hinders development.

Overcoming the Fear of Change

If you have BPD, you're likely to have some concerns about seeking treatment and making life changes. These are normal, acceptable, and expected fears. If you feel that your therapist is pushing you too hard to make changes, then openly discuss your fears. You two should build a mutual game plan to tackle these issues at a speed that works for you.

Losing who you are: Many people with BPD are grappling with questions about who they are, what they value, where they belong in the world, and what their long-term interests are all about. Not infrequently, individuals with BPD in their self-concept accept only one part of themselves— their condition. They may not like BPD, but they believe they are defined by the diagnosis. Because of that belief, they worry that losing BPD might leave them with no identity whatsoever. Imagine going through each day with no idea of who you are or what your life is all about — a rather scary thought, right?

Opening up: No need for cold feet. As people with BPD think about their childhoods, they sometimes recall being constantly scolded in their lives by parents or other important people. Such people were telling them they shouldn't do, say, or feel what they did, do, and felt. Therapists aren't there to recreate the role that people from childhood have played. Instead, they accept all sentiments as legitimate and valid. Therapy can help you control your emotions and assist you in making changes—and it does so in a healthy environment. You can begin by saying, "I feel very scared to disclose to you the real me." Your therapist would probably say something encouraging or welcoming in response.

Dreading even more loss: Don't assess those who want to support because people with BPD suffer childhood loss, trauma, abuse, or neglect. As adults, the erratic moods and impulsiveness that they developed during childhood will lead to loss of friends, family, and loves. As a consequence, with a combination of fear and hope, they look at new relationships; they desire closeness but expect abandonment. Starting treatment involves engaging with another person in a therapeutic relationship, which can be an extremely frightening idea for someone who has been part of numerous hurtful relationships. Individuals with BPD frequently misbehave in social situations to defend against fearful abandonment. They feel rejecting others is better than rejection. Therefore, they test people's limits and patience that try to help them make sure they do the hurt— not the other way around. Those with BPD often commonly check their relationships with significant others and therapists.

Taking Charge and Giving Up the Victim Role

People are seeking answers to why bad things happen to them— they are trying to find out who to blame or what to blame for. Similarly, many people with BPD want to know why they have the disorder, and who can blame them for it. Sadly, typically this search for a culprit ends up causing more harm than good. BPD is not responsible for any single cause, and no one is to blame.

When you've undergone a trauma, it's completely natural to feel rage at the person or people you claim to harm. You have to remember, however, that your rage shackles you to your past— you get trapped in the midst of the old trauma. Sometimes people with BPD think forgiving means somehow admitting that what happened to them was acceptable. But learning to let go is not saying that what happened was all right; it is saying you are willing to heal. If you're dealing with BPD, try to understand that although you're not to blame for your BPD, it's up to you to make the improvements you want in your life.

Getting comfortable with the Change process

Beginning therapy can feel like a difficult and risky decision. You don't know what to expect, and you're worried you might not get any better. Change takes time and varies in progress. Remember learning how to ride a bike as a kid? You got off to a lot of help. Then you had to hang on to training wheels or someone else, or you fall over. You slowly learned to walk with assistance on two wheels. Then the training wheels come off, or they let the individual go. You were alone for a second or two. Balanced for only a short time, the wheels began wobbling, and you once again needed some extra help. Learning to ride a bike takes repeated trials and many drops on most kids. The juggling is too appalling and too complex for some people. They can give up in just a few months or even a year, just to try again. A couple of kids have so much trouble they never know how to ride a bike. Yet, fortunately, most children stay with it long enough to learn how to ride without any assistance. The common saying that you'll never forget once you learn how to ride a bike is true. Even so, with a little apprehension, most adults who have not been on a bike since childhood start slowly but quickly recover their abilities.

Getting help with BPD (like most problems in life) is much like learning how to ride a bike. You need a whole lot of support at first. In the beginning, you can fail and fall quite a bit. You could even give up for some time. Yet, in the end, most people who stick with either bike riding or psychotherapy develop skills and discipline. They still wobble from time to time and even fall off sometimes, but the skills become second nature to them with repeated practice. Like riding a bike, you'll never forget after learning how to cope with your problems — sure you might be scared and start slowly, but with a little support, you can get back up straight again.

CPSIA information can be obtained
at www.ICGtesting.com
Printed in the USA
BVHW042027060322
630780BV00012B/222